# Recipes for Fas Metabolism

Food-Based Ways to Boost Your Metabolism

by

Josephine Ellise

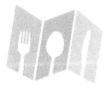

# Copyright Notices

# Table of Contents

# Introduction

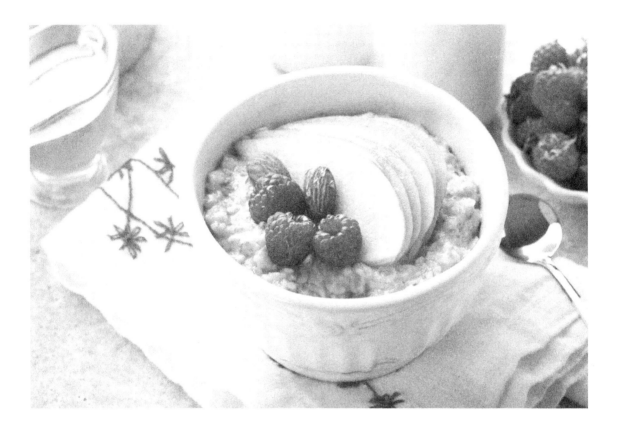

Are you prepared to start a diet that lets you consume as much food as you want while still losing weight? I'm glad you're here, Fast Metabolism Diet! With this diet, you can eat a lot without keeping track of your calories, grams, or food categories, or even without denying yourself dessert. That is correct! It's more about carefully alternating the various dietary categories each week rather than being vegan or even carb-free. Your body will then experience a number of physiological changes as a result of which your metabolism will be greatly increased.

The Fast Metabolism plan in *"Recipes for Fast Metabolism"* largely consists of three steps, including:

Phase I: Eating primarily carbohydrates and fruits (usually Monday-Tuesday)

Phase II: Eating mostly protein and veggies (usually Wednesday-Thursday)

Phase III: Integrating healthy oils and fats into your diet (usually Friday-Sunday)

Athletes, famous people, and those recuperating from chronic diseases have all found success with this regimen for weight loss and general health improvement. This is the moment for you to follow suit. Let's explore a few recipes that might get you started on the correct path to Fast Metabolism.

xxxxxxxxxxxxxxxxxxxxxxxxxxxxxxxxxxxxxxxxxxxxxxx

# 1. Honey Mustard Chicken Drumsticks

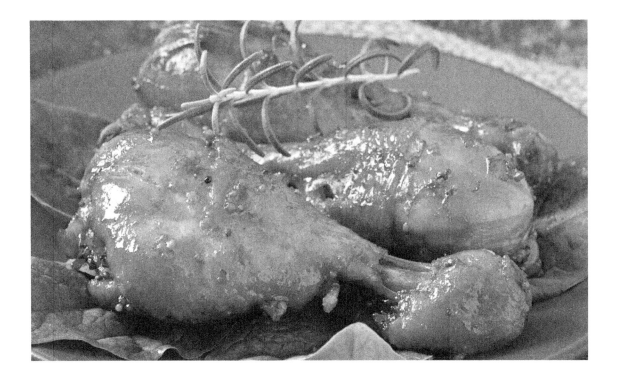

**Makes:** 6

**Total Prep Time:** 1 Hour 30 Minutes

**Ingredient List:**

- 3 lbs. drumsticks
- 4 oz. flour
- 1 teaspoon salt
- ½ teaspoons paprika
- 1 teaspoon white pepper
- ½ teaspoons chicken seasoning
- ½ cup soft margarine
- ½ cup honey
- ½ cup mustard
- 6 teaspoons lime juice
- ½ teaspoons salt

xxxxxxxxxxxxxxxxxxxxxxxxxxxxxxxxxxxxxxxxxxxxx

**Procedure:**

A. Wash and drain drumsticks. Use a clean cloth or paper towel to dry the

B. In a paper bag, combine salt, almond flour, paprika, chicken seasoning, and white pepper.

C. Put chicken in a bag and shake vigorously to coat properly. Melt margarine in a baking pan, and roll pieces of chicken in melted margarine until all sides are coated.

D. Fix the chicken pieces, skin side down in the baking pan, packing them close to each other but not overcrowded.

E. Bake at 400°F for 30 minutes. Turn the chicken pieces over and pour on the

F. Bake for a further 20 minutes or until cooked. Set aside.

G. Mix all the ingredients listed together and pour over the chicken and serve.

# 2. Crepe Fettuccine with Tomatoes, Fresh Mozzarella and Pesto

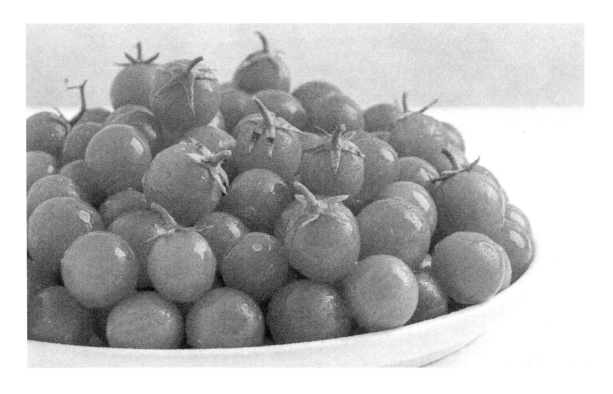

**Makes:** 6-8

**Total Prep Time:** 1 Hour and 50 Minutes

**Ingredient List:**

- All-purpose ricotta crepes (15, see recipe)
- Olive oil (2 tablespoons)
- Assorted fresh cherry tomatoes (1 lb., cut into halves and quarters)
- Red chili flakes (1/2 teaspoons, crushed)
- Fresh mozzarella (1 lb., removed from the water and cubed)
- Parmesan cheese (1/4 cup cheese, grated)
- Fresh basil (16 leaves)
- Pesto sauce (1 tbsp)
- Salt and fresh cracked pepper, to taste

xxxxxxxxxxxxxxxxxxxxxxxxxxxxxxxxxxxxxxxxxxxxxxxxx

**Procedure:**

A. Put the crepes in small stacks of 5; roll them into little tight logs. Slice crepe into ½" sizes. Put aside.
B. Heat the oil in a suitable-sized sauté pan, on medium flame.
C. When hot, add assorted tomatoes, chili flakes, and a pinch of pepper and salt. Sauté for 60 secs.
D. Add in pesto and noodles and mix until well coated. Cook for 60 secs.
E. Stir in mozzarella and cook until the cheese starts melting.
F. Add the fresh mozzarella and toss. Shared in 4 portions.
G. Use fresh basil and parmesan cheese to garnish. Serve!

# 3. Buffalo "Potato" Wedges with Blue Cheese Drizzle

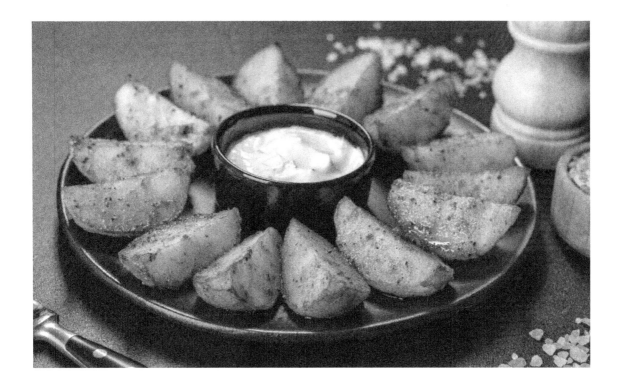

**Makes:** 4

**Total Time:** 1 Hour

**Ingredient List:**

- Rutabagas (2 medium, cleaned and peeled)
- Butter (4 tablespoons)
- Salt (1/2 tsp)
- Onion powder (1/2 teaspoons)
- Black pepper (1/8 teaspoons)
- Buffalo wing sauce (1/2 cup)
- Blue cheese dressing (1/4 cup)
- Green onions (2, chopped)

xxxxxxxxxxxxxxxxxxxxxxxxxxxxxxxxxxxxxxxxxxxxxxxx

**Procedure:**

A. Heat the oven to 400°F and use parchment paper to line a baking tray.

B. Wash and peel the rutabagas. Clean and peel rutabagas and cut them into a wedge shape.

C. On low heat, melt butter and stir in onion powder, salt, onion, and black pepper.

D. Use seasoned melted butter to coat wedge-shaped rutabaga liberally.

E. Arrange the layers singly on a baking sheet. Bake for half an hour.

F. Remove for a short while from the oven; coat in buffalo wing sauce. Return to the oven and bake for a further 15 mins.

G. Place wedges on a serving plate and trickle with blue cheese dressing. Garnish with chopped green onion on top. Serve.

# 4. Chocolate Chia Pudding

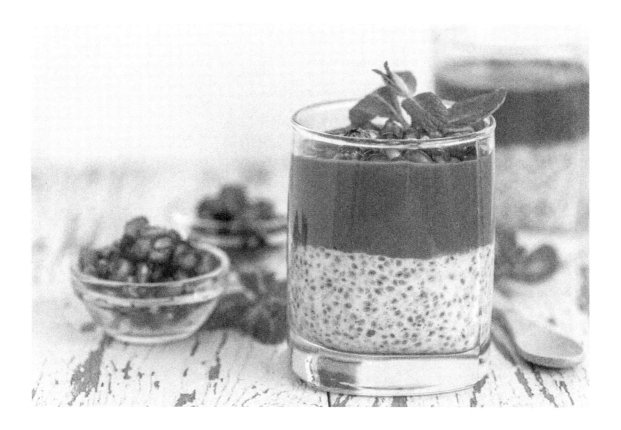

**Makes:** 2

**Total Prep Time:** 8 Hours 5 Minutes

**Ingredient List:**

- Almond milk (1¼ cup)
- Chia seeds (1/4 cup)
- Cacao powder (1½ tablespoons, raw)
- Stevia (1/4 teaspoons, liquid)
- Cacao nibs (raw, enough to garnish)

xxxxxxxxxxxxxxxxxxxxxxxxxxxxxxxxxxxxxxxxxxxxxxx

**Procedure:**

A. Add your cacao powder, chia seeds, stevia, and almond milk to a bowl, and whisk to combine until no lumps remain.
B. Cover tightly and place in the refrigerator to set overnight.
C. Top with cacao nibs and serve.

# 5. Garlic Gnocchi

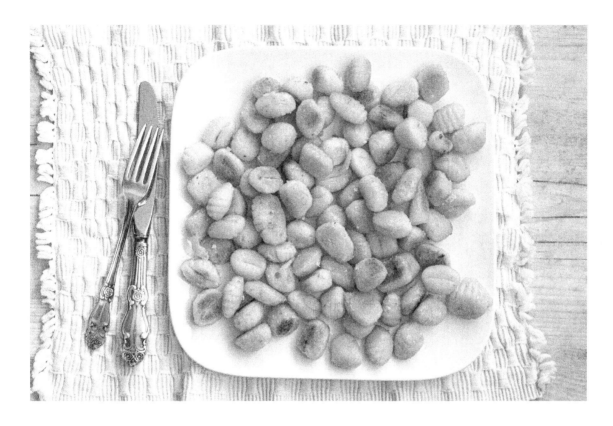

**Makes:** 2

**Total Time:** 25 Minutes

**Ingredient List:**

- Kraft Low-Moisture Part-Skim mozzarella (2 cups shredded. If this particular cheese is not used, it will fall apart when boiling.)
- Egg yolks (3)
- Granulated garlic (1 teaspoon)
- Butter olive oil for sautéing

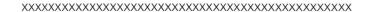

xxxxxxxxxxxxxxxxxxxxxxxxxxxxxxxxxxxxxxxxxxxxxxxxxx

**Procedure:**

A. Combine cheese and garlic in a microwavable bowl. Use the microwave to melt the Give it a time period of 1-1 ½ mins.

B. Fold in egg yolks individually until a consistent dough is formed (this actually takes some effort).

C. Divide dough into 4 balls. Put it in the refrigerator for at least 10 minutes.

D. Grease your hands and a piece of parchment paper lightly and roll each ball into a 15" log. Slice the log into 1" pieces (gnocchi).

E. Boil half a gallon of water in a large pot. Put all the gnocchi into the pot and cook until they are afloat. This takes about 3 mins.

F. Use a colander to strain off the

G. On a medium-high flame, heat a suitable size non-stick pan.

H. Pour a tablespoons of olive oil in the pan and add a tablespoon of butter.

I. Place gnocchi in the pan and sauté each side until golden brown.

J. Add salt and pepper to taste. Serve!

# 6. Root Beer Ribs

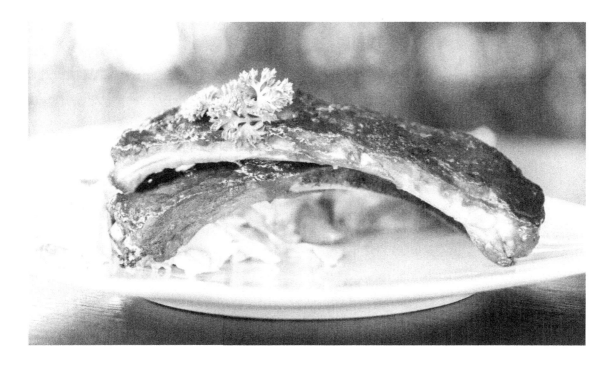

**Makes:** 3-4

**Total Time:** 2 Hours 30 Minutes

**Ingredient List:**

- Pork spare ribs (2 lbs.)

**For the rub:**

- Salt (1 tsp)
- Pepper (1 tsp)
- Spicy Hungarian paprika (1 tsp)

**For the braise:**

- Large red onion, minced (1)
- Section ginger, peeled, minced (1")
- Cumin, crushed (1 tsp)
- Spicy Hungarian paprika (1/4 tsp)
- Bay leaves (3)
- Cinnamon (1/4 tsp)
- Root beer (1 bottle, 12 ounces)
- Beef or chicken broth (1 cup)
- Rosemary (2 sprigs)
- Thyme (3 sprigs)

xxxxxxxxxxxxxxxxxxxxxxxxxxxxxxxxxxxxxxxxxxxxxxxxxxx

**Procedure:**

A.  Set your oven to preheat to 275°F. As well, your large Dutch oven should be heated over a high fire. Your rib back should be rubbed in with salt, pepper, and your spicy paprika mix.

B.  Sear the ribs all over using a cooking tong until it gets to a good golden brown.

C.  Now remove your ribs to a plate. Your Dutch oven should be cleared of all the oil now but leave behind 2 tablespoons where onion should be added to medium-high heat until soft and the edges become brown.

D.  Return your ribs to the pot, including with it all the braise ingredients listed, and boil the entire mixture. For a little while, cover it before placing it in the oven.

E.  While in the oven and turning the ribs halfway through, braise them for about 2 1/2 – 3 hours before removing them from the oven.

F.  A large skillet should be placed on low heat for which you will now place your ribs. For the Dutch oven, place your burner on high heat and remove the bay leaves.

G.  Boil the sauce down in here for approximately 20 minutes until you get to the desired thickness. Glaze your ribs with a bit of the sauce while stirring it.

H.  Finely slice your ribs nicely and smother them with sauce. Serve and enjoy over rice, polenta, or potatoes.

# 7. Stuffed Eggplant

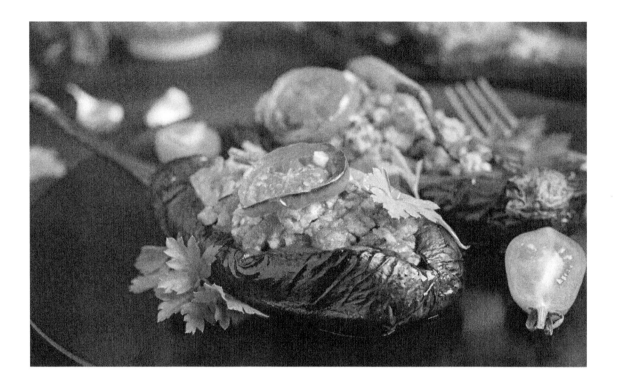

**Makes:** 6

**Total Time:** 1 Hour 35 Minutes

**Ingredient List:**

- Eggplants (6 slender, preferably Japanese eggplants)
- Olive oil (4 tablespoons, divided)
- Red onions (2 medium, chopped)
- Garlic (4 cloves, minced)
- Fresh parsley (3 tablespoons, chopped)
- Bell pepper (1 green, seeded, and chopped)
- Tomatoes (4, chopped)
- Raw coconut palm sugar (1 teaspoon)
- Ground cumin (1 teaspoon)
- Tomato paste (1 tablespoon)
- Salt (to taste)
- Black pepper (to taste)

xxxxxxxxxxxxxxxxxxxxxxxxxxxxxxxxxxxxxxxxxxxxxxx

**Procedure:**

A.  Place a rack in the middle of the oven and preheat to 450°F

B.  Use aluminum foil or parchment paper to line the baking tray then brush it with some olive oil.

C.  Remove the wide strips from the skin of the eggplants. A vegetable peeler should be used.

D.  Use a vegetable peeler to remove wide strips of the eggplants' skin. Split the eggplants in a lengthwise direction, careful not to slice straight through them.

E.  In each eggplant, sprinkle a generous pinch of salt, and leave them in a colander to rest for about half an hour.

F.  Place eggplants on the lined baking tray, and bake for 20 minutes or until the outer skin begins shriveling.

G.  When completed, remove and set aside. Set a skillet over medium heat, add 2 tablespoons of oil and onions then sauté until soft.

H.  Add the bell pepper and garlic. Continue cooking for another 10 mins., until the vegetables are soft.

I.  Use salt and pepper to season, and mix in the sugar, chopped tomato, cumin, parsley, and tomato paste, and parsley.

J.  Cook for 5 mins, until the fragrance permeates the air. Set aside.

# 8. Broccoli Crust Pizza

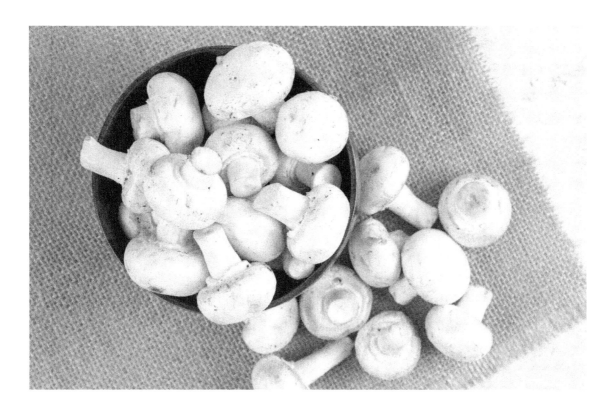

**Makes:** 2

**Total Time:** 35 Minutes

**Ingredient List:**

- Mushrooms (3 large, sliced)
- Onion (2 small, minced)
- Carrots (2 cubed)
- Turnip (1 small, cubed)
- Chayote (1, cubed)
- Celery (2 stalks, cubed)
- Tin corn (1- 14 oz)
- Garlic (4 cloves, diced)
- Ginger (2 inches, crushed)
- Bay leaves (3)
- Turmeric (1/4 teaspoons)
- Black pepper (1 teaspoon)
- 1 pinch of salt

xxxxxxxxxxxxxxxxxxxxxxxxxxxxxxxxxxxxxxxxxxxxxxxxx

**Procedure:**

A. Heat your oven to 392°F. Pulse the onion and broccoli in a food mixer until chopped finely.

B. Add the balance of ingredients listedand pulse until all are chopped and thoroughly combined. Put aside the mixture for 15 mins.. This will allow the liquid to be absorbed by the chia seeds and husk.

C. Use your fingers or a roller to form the pizza on a baking tray covered with parchment paper.

D. Spread pizza in the same thickness right around, so it bakes evenly. Bake for a 10-minute period then flip it gently over and bake for a further 5 mins.

E. Remove the pizza crust from the oven and add the desired topping. Here are some suggestions: organic tomato puree, chili powder, a small amount of garlic powder, fresh basil, goat cheese, paprika, sliced tomato, and onion rings.

F. Bake pizzas for an additional 5 mins. then remove. Add arugula and a little fresher basil and serve.

# 9. Sliced Apple Almond Butter

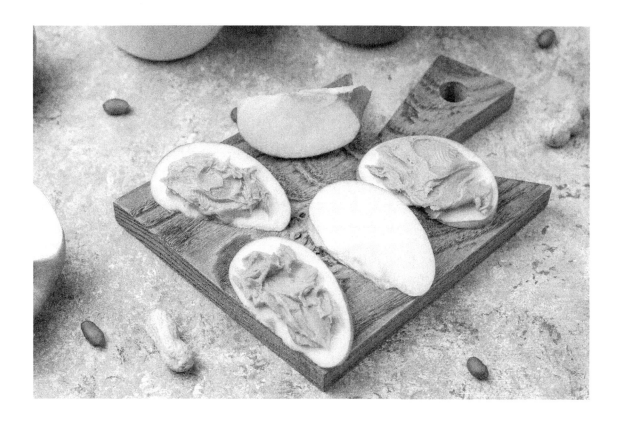

**Makes:** 1

**Total Time:** 5 Minutes

**Ingredient List:**

- Apple (2, Granny Smith)
- Almond Butter (2 tablespoons)

xxxxxxxxxxxxxxxxxxxxxxxxxxxxxxxxxxxxxxxxxxxxxxxxx

**Procedure:**

A. Prepare your apple, by breaking the stem and then slicing it to discard the seeds and core.
B. Slice your apples into thin slices and lay them flat on a serving plate.
C. Top with drizzles of almond butter and enjoy!

# 10. Beef Stew

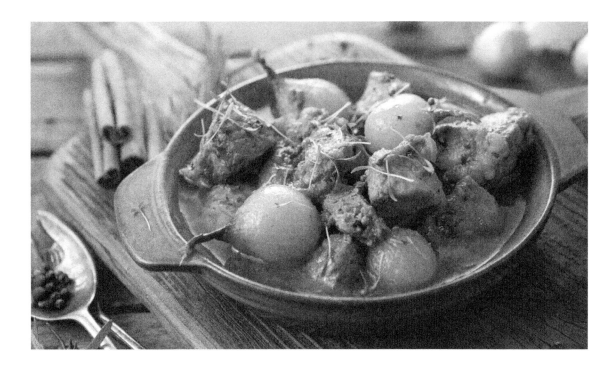

**Makes:** 3-4

**Total Time:** 2 Hours

**Ingredient List:**

- Onion (1, small, diced)
- Carrot (1, small, diced)
- Celery (1 stalk, diced)
- Thyme (1 sprig)
- Bay Leaf (1 dry)
- Cloves (2, whole)
- Beef Stock (3 Cups)
- Stew Beef (2 lbs., trimmed, diced)
- Sea salt and pepper (1 tsp each)
- Vegetable oil (1/2 Cup)
- Tomato Paste (1 tablespoon)
- White Wine (1 Cup, dry)
- Parsley (3 Tablespoons, chopped)
- Lemon Zest (1 tablespoon)

xxxxxxxxxxxxxxxxxxxxxxxxxxxxxxxxxxxxxxxxxxxxxxxx

**Procedure:**

A. Create a bouquet garni by tying your cheesecloth with the thyme, rosemary, cloves, and bay leaf cloves inside then secure it with a piece of twine.

B. Use a piece of paper towel to remove the excess moisture from the beef pieces in a patting motion.

C. Season with pepper and salt. Heat the oil in your Dutch oven pot until it begins to smoke.

D. Place the beef to brown on all sides. Take the beef off the heat and set aside.

E. In the pot, you took the beef pieces from, pour in the carrots, onion, and celery then add salt to the

F. Sauté for about 8 minutes or until completely soft.

G. Mix the tomato paste with the carrot mixture in the pot and add browned beef.

H. Pour in the white wine and allow it to cook until the liquid has been reduced by half.

I. Pour in the 2 cups of the beef stock along with the bouquet garni and allow it to boil.

J. Cover the pot, set the heat to low, and simmer until the meat is literally falling off the bone when lifted. Ensure that the liquid is about ¾ way up the shank by checking on it in 15-minute intervals.

K. When the meat has cooked, remove the beef from the pot and plate it in preparation to serve.

L. Remove and discard the kitchen twine and the bouquet garni. Use the juices from the pot to pour over the beef pieces.

M. Serve and Enjoy!

# 11. Turkey Burgers with Corn

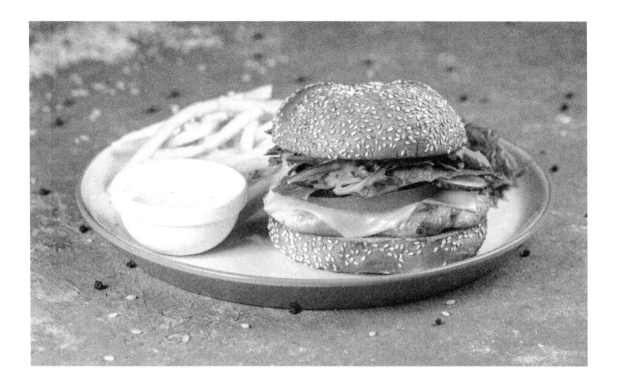

**Makes:** 1

**Total Time:** 50 Minutes

**Ingredient List:**

**Burger mix:**

- Turkey mince (111g)
- Egg (1, beaten)
- Spring onion (1 tablespoon, chopped)
- Garlic (1 clove, minced)
- Chili Pepper (1/2 tsp, ground)
- Vegetables
- Corn on the cob (1, medium, warmed)

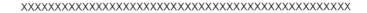

**Procedure:**

A. Add all your burger ingredients listedto a large bowl, and gently massage to combine.
B. Set to marinate in the refrigerator for at least 30 minutes.
C. Split your mixture evenly in half, and form into 2 burger patties.
D. Cook on a preheated grill until fully cooked (about 5 min per side).
E. Serve alongside corn on the cob.

# 12. Hummus and Crudités

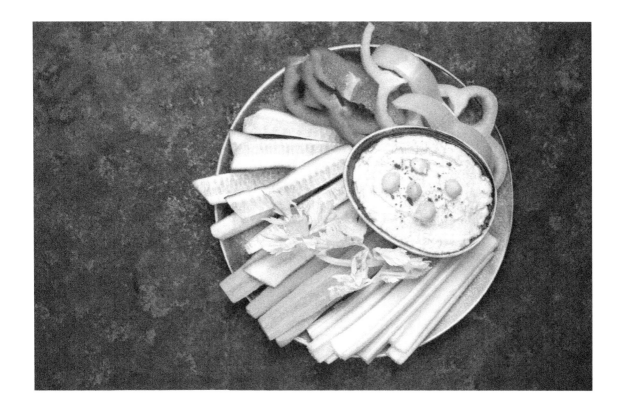

**Makes:** 1

**Total Prep Time:** 10 Minutes

**Ingredient List:**

- Hummus (40 grams)
- Carrots (3 jumbos, cut into small sticks)
- Cucumber (1/2 cup, cut into small sticks)
- Red Bell Pepper (1/2 cup, cut into small sticks)

xxxxxxxxxxxxxxxxxxxxxxxxxxxxxxxxxxxxxxxxxxxxxx

**Procedure:**

A. Add your hummus to a small bowl and set it in the center of a serving plate.
B. Add your veggies around the hummus and enjoy!

# 13. Smoked BBQ Beans

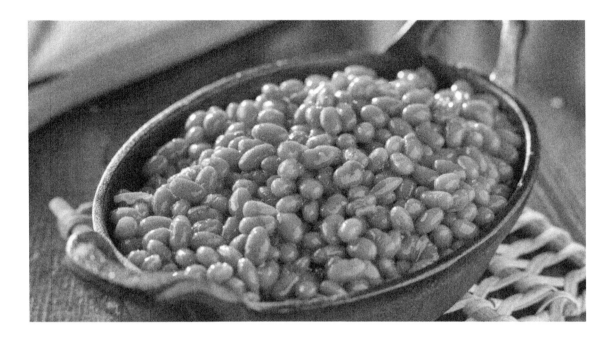

**Makes:** 3-4

**Total Prep Time:** 1 Hour

**Ingredient List:**

- Bacon (center cut, 5 slices, chopped)
- Yellow Onion (1, chopped)
- Garlic Cloves (5, minced)
- Jalapeno (1, chopped)
- Pinto (1 lb.)
- Water (6 Cups)
- BBQ Sauce (1 Cup)
- Spicy Brown Mustard (2 Tablespoons)
- Adobo Sauce (2 Tablespoons, from canned Chipotles)
- Tabasco Sauce (2 Tablespoons, smoked)
- Molasses (2 Tablespoons)
- Guinness (splash, optional)
- Salt (2 Tsp)
- Pepper (1 tsp)

xxxxxxxxxxxxxxxxxxxxxxxxxxxxxxxxxxxxxxxxxxxxxx

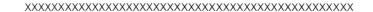

**Procedure:**

A. Prepare your beans (wash, sort, and soak) overnight. Set your Dutch oven to preheat on the top of the stove.

B. Add the bacon to the heated oven and allow it to brown until crisp. At this point, add the jalapeno and onions then proceed to sauté until the onions become soft.

C. Continue to sauté while you add the garlic. Continue for about a minute.

D. Pour in the beans, and water then cover and allow it to cook on low to medium heat for about an hour or until the beans become soft.

E. Add a bit of your preferred BBQ sauce along with the brown sugar, adobo sauce, Tabasco, mustard salt, and pepper while stirring well.

F. Remove the cover and allow it to simmer until the sauce thickens and the beans become completely cooked (should be about an hour).

G. Serve and enjoy.

# 14. Oats Porridge

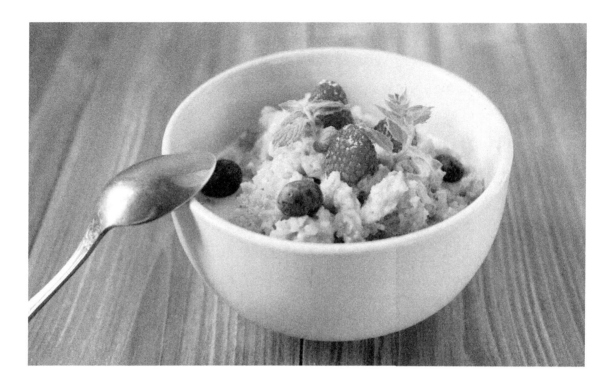

**Makes:** 1

**Total Prep Time:** 10 Minutes

**Ingredient List:**

- Quaker Oats (40g)
- Milk (180 ml, 1%)

xxxxxxxxxxxxxxxxxxxxxxxxxxxxxxxxxxxxxxxxxxxxxxxxxx

**Procedure:**

A. Add your milk to a small saucepan over medium heat, and allow it to come to a boil, while stirring.
B. Add oats, stir, and lower your heat so that the mixture just simmers.
C. Allow it to simmer, stirring occasionally, until your milk becomes mostly absorbed (about 2 additional minutes).

# 15. Smoked Salmon Eggs in Endive

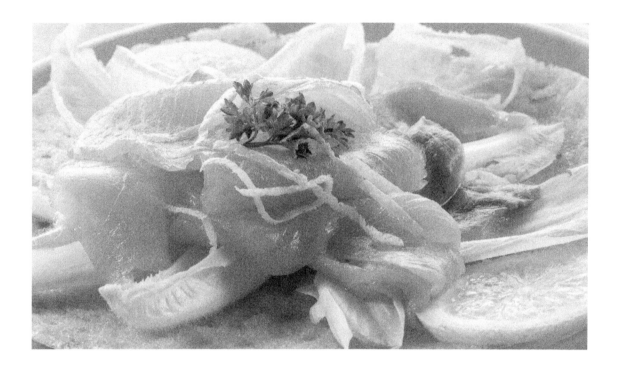

**Makes:** 2

**Total Prep Time:** 20 Minutes

**Ingredient List:**

- Eggs (4, hard-cooked, chopped finely)
- Dill Pickle (1 tablespoon, minced)
- Chives (1 tablespoon, chopped)
- Endive leaves (8)
- Salmon (4 oz., smoked, sliced)

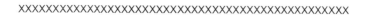

**Procedure:**

A. Add the chives, pickles, and eggs to a medium bowl, then stir to combine.

B. Lay your endive leaves on a flat surface and spoon your mixture evenly into your 8 leaves.

C. Add some smoked salmon to the top of each egg scoop and serve. Enjoy!

# 16. Parmesan Fried Eggplant

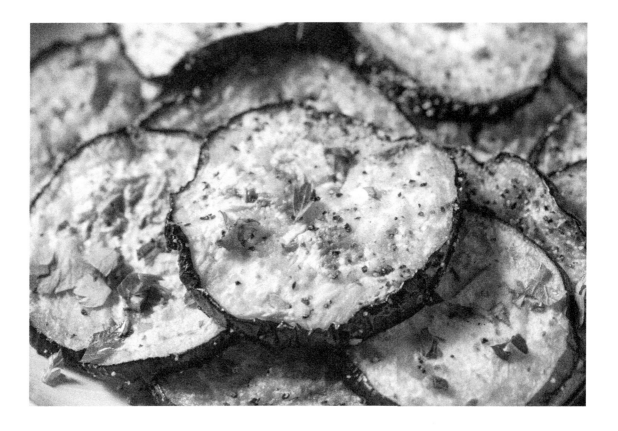

**Makes:** 6

**Total Prep Time:** 21 Minutes

**Ingredient List:**

- Eggplant (1 medium)
- Salt (1/2 teaspoons)
- Egg (1 large)
- Almond flour (1 cup)
- Parmesan cheese (1 cup, grated)
- Garlic powder (2 teaspoons)
- Salt (to taste)
- Pepper (to taste)
- Coconut oil (1/4 cup)

xxxxxxxxxxxxxxxxxxxxxxxxxxxxxxxxxxxxxxxxxxxxxxxxxx

**Procedure:**

A. Prepare eggplant by slicing it into thick slices. Lay your slices on a flat surface then blot with a hand towel to remove excess water.

B. Season with salt and allow to marinate for about 30 minutes. Blot, once more to remove any water that may have pooled up. Blot eggplant dry with a paper towel.

C. Add eggs to a medium bowl and whisk until well beaten.

D. Add garlic powder, parmesan cheese, and almond flour to a large bowl.

E. Season with pepper, and salt, and stir to combine.

F. Set a skillet with coconut oil to get hot, over medium heat.

G. Add your eggplant slices to your egg bowl.

H. Use a pair of tongs to lift out, gently shake off any excess egg drippings, then dredge into flour mixture.

I. Lift out and add to the hot skillet to fry until browned on all sides and crispy.

J. Repeat the process until all your eggplant has been cooked. Enjoy!

# 17. Hot Green Beans and Noodle Soup

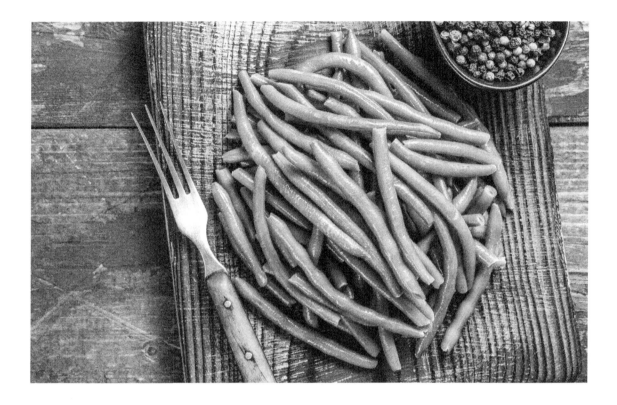

**Makes:** 3

**Total Prep Time:** 1hr 40min

**Ingredient List:**

- 1 cup green beans, boiled
- 1 package of noodles, boiled
- 2 cups chicken broth
- ½ cup shredded chicken, boiled
- 1 tablespoon lemon juice
- 2 tablespoons apple cider vinegar
- 1 tablespoon soya sauce
- 2 tablespoons chili garlic sauce
- 4-5 garlic cloves, minced
- ½ teaspoons black pepper
- ¼ teaspoons salt
- 1 tablespoon oil

xxxxxxxxxxxxxxxxxxxxxxxxxxxxxxxxxxxxxxxxxxxxxxx

**Procedure:**

A. Heat oil in a pan, add onion and garlic cloves and cook for 1 minute. Add all red beans and chicken, and fry for 5 minutes.

B. Add chicken broth, soya sauce, chili garlic sauce, vinegar, salt, and pepper, and mix well. Leave to cook on medium heat for 10 minutes.

C. Stir in noodles and cook for another 5 minutes.

D. Ladle into serving bowls. Drizzle lemon juice on top. Serve and enjoy.

# 18. Egg Stuffed Avocado

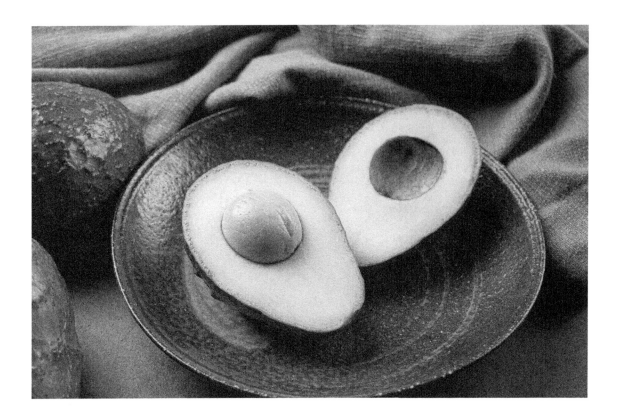

**Makes:** 2

**Total Prep Time:** 15 Minutes

**Ingredient List:**

- Avocado (1 extra-large, seeded)
- Eggs (4 large, free-range)
- Mayonnaise (¼ cup)
- Sour cream (2 tablespoons)
- Dijon mustard (1 teaspoon)
- Spring onions (2 medium)
- Salt (to taste)
- Black pepper (to taste)

xxxxxxxxxxxxxxxxxxxxxxxxxxxxxxxxxxxxxxxxxxxxxxxx

**Procedure:**

A. Set a small saucepan with enough water to fill ¾ of the pan. Season water with salt and allow it to come to a boil.

B. Gently add your eggs to your boiling water with a spoon. Allow eggs to cook for about 10 minutes to achieve a hard-boiled egg.

C. Switch off the heat and carefully transfer your eggs to a bowl of iced water with a slotted spoon. Allow to cool down.

D. Once cool, peel the shell from the eggs.

E. Dice your eggs and add to a medium bowl. Scoop out about a tablespoons of avocado flesh from the center of each half, dice, and add to eggs.

F. Add spring onions, sour cream, Dijon mustard, and mayo. Season to taste with pepper, and salt. Stir to combine.

G. Spoon the mixture evenly back into your avocado halves. Serve, and enjoy!

# 19. Pesto Scrambled Eggs

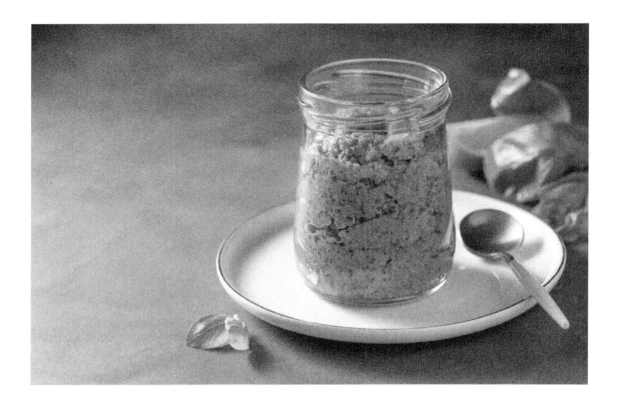

**Makes:** 1

**Total Prep Time:** 10 Minutes

**Ingredient List:**

- Eggs (3 large, free-range)
- Butter (1 tablespoon)
- Pesto (1 tablespoon)
- Crème fraiche (2 tablespoons)
- Salt (to taste)
- Black pepper (to taste)

xxxxxxxxxxxxxxxxxxxxxxxxxxxxxxxxxxxxxxxxxxxxxxxx

**Procedure:**

A. Add your eggs to a mixing bowl then season with salt and pepper. Whisk until fully beaten (should be frothy).

B. Next, set a skillet, over low heat, with your butter, and allow it to melt. Once melted, add eggs, stir, and continue to cook while stirring over low heat.

C. Stir in your pesto then remove from heat. Add the Crème Fraiche and stir well to fully incorporate.

D. Serve with avocados or buns!

# 20. Banana Pumpkin Almond Cake

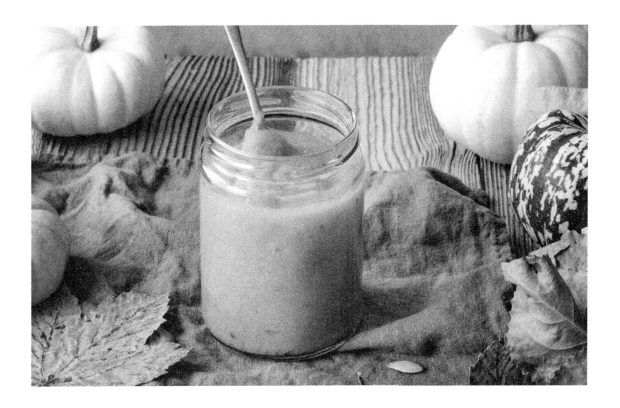

**Makes:** 12

**Total Prep Time:** 1hr 40min

**Ingredient List:**

- 1 lb. coconut sugar
- 6 tablespoons butter
- 1 lb. almond flour
- 4 teaspoons baking powder
- 1 teaspoon salt
- ½ cup banana, mashed
- 1/2 cup pumpkin puree
- 1 teaspoon Cinnamon
- ¼ teaspoons nutmeg
- 1 pint. evaporated milk

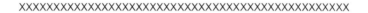

xxxxxxxxxxxxxxxxxxxxxxxxxxxxxxxxxxxxxxxxxxxxxxxxxx

**Procedure:**

A. Grease and line a 10 in. Bundt pan. Preheat the oven to 325°F.

B. Combine the almond flour, baking powder, and salt. Lay aside.

C. Cream 1 lb. of sugar and 6 tablespoons butter until really fluffy in a large container.

D. Fold in the flour mixture, and alternate with the evaporated milk.

E. Mix in the cranberries and pour the mixture into a greased

F. Bake in the prepared oven for an hour.

G. When the cake is baked, a toothpick inserted should come out clean.

H. Allow 10 mins. for cooling then turn it out on a wire rack, and let it remain until totally cooled.

I. Serve and enjoy.

# 21. Baked Zucchini Fries

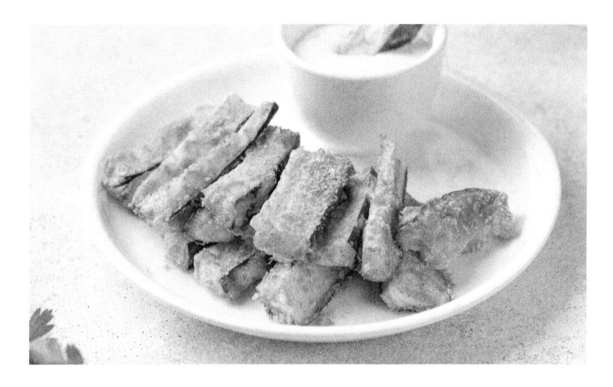

**Makes:** 2

**Total Prep Time:** 8 Minutes

**Ingredient List:**

- Zucchini (6, cut like fries)
- Paprika (1 tsp)
- Garlic powder (1/2 tsp)
- Oregano (1/4 tsp)
- Oil (1 tablespoon)
- Salt (1/4 teaspoons)
- Pepper (1/4 teaspoons)

xxxxxxxxxxxxxxxxxxxxxxxxxxxxxxxxxxxxxxxxxxxxxxxx

**Procedure:**

A. Set your oven to 390°F.
B. Toss all your ingredients listed in a large bowl and add to a lined baking tray in a single layer.
C. Allow baking for 5 - 7 minutes (your basil should be crisp in texture). Serve and enjoy!

# 22. Eggs Florentine

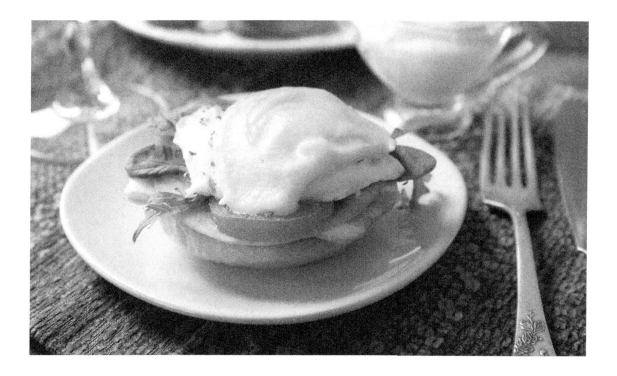

**Makes:** 1

**Total Prep Time:** 8 Minutes

**Ingredient List:**

- 2 large eggs (2 large)
- Extra virgin olive oil (1 tablespoon, unfiltered)
- An egg fast alfredo sauce (5 tablespoons)
- Organic Parmigiano Reggiano wedge (1 tablespoon, divided)
- Organic baby spinach (3 grams)
- Red pepper flakes (1 pinch)

xxxxxxxxxxxxxxxxxxxxxxxxxxxxxxxxxxxxxxxxxxxxxxxx

**Procedure:**

A. Set the oven rack in the top groove nearest to the broiler. Set the broiler to a preheat se

B. Place olive oil in a non-stick skillet and put it to heat over medium-high

C. Gently, fry eggs over medium flame, until egg whites are opaque but the yolk is still runny. This takes roughly 4 mins. Do not turn over eggs.

D. Prepare the casserole in the meantime. Dribble some olive oil in each casserole container or spray with cooking spray (olive oil).

E. In the bottom of the casserole, spread half of the Alfredo sauce. Slide gently, the half-done egg atop the

F. Spread leftover Alfredo sauce and half of the parmesan cheese over the

G. Set the casserole under the broiler and broil for 2-3 mins or until the eggs have formed and the top has bubbly golden spots.

H. Remove from broiler and top with thinly sliced (julienne) baby spinach leaves, unused Parmesan cheese, and a dash of red pepper flakes.

I. Serve instantly.

# 23. Banana Low-Fat Yogurt

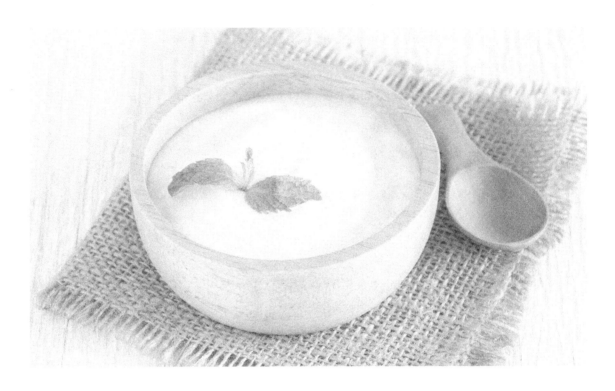

**Makes:** 1

**Total Prep Time:** 5 Minutes

**Ingredient List:**

- Yogurt (100 grams, low–fat)
- Banana (1)
- Cinnamon (1/4 teaspoons)

xxxxxxxxxxxxxxxxxxxxxxxxxxxxxxxxxxxxxxxxxxxxxxxx

**Procedure:**

A. Combine all of your ingredients listed in your blender, and process until smooth. Enjoy!

# 24.. Slow Cooker Roasted Red Bell Pepper Soup

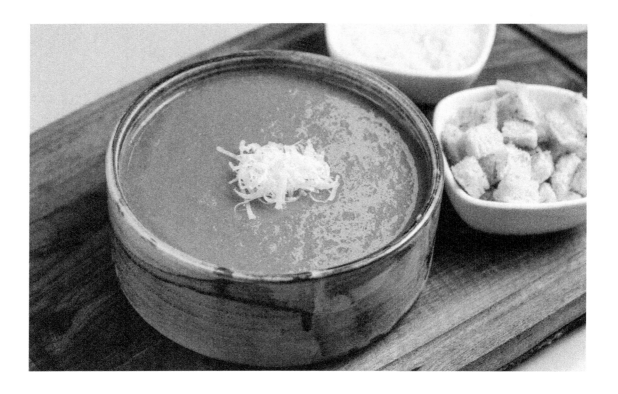

**Makes:** 4

**Total Prep Time:** 8 Hours 15 Minutes

**Ingredient List:**

- 1 cup roasted red bell pepper, chopped
- 1 teaspoon ginger paste
- 1 small onion, chopped
- 2 cups vegetable broth
- 2 tablespoons vinegar
- 1 lemon, sliced
- 1 green chili, chopped
- 4-5 garlic cloves, minced
- ½ teaspoons black pepper
- ¼ teaspoons salt
- 1 tablespoon oil

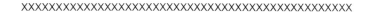

xxxxxxxxxxxxxxxxxxxxxxxxxxxxxxxxxxxxxxxxxxxxxxx

**Procedure:**

B. Heat oil in a saucepan, add ginger paste, and cook for 1 minute.

C. Add red bell peppers and fry well for 5-10 minutes.

D. Now add onions, salt, pepper, vinegar, green chilies, and lemon slices and mix well.

E. Remove from heat and add to a slow cooker. Add vegetable broth and leave to cook on low for 8 hours.

F. Spoon into serving bowls. Serve and enjoy.

# 25. Leek Mushroom Frittata

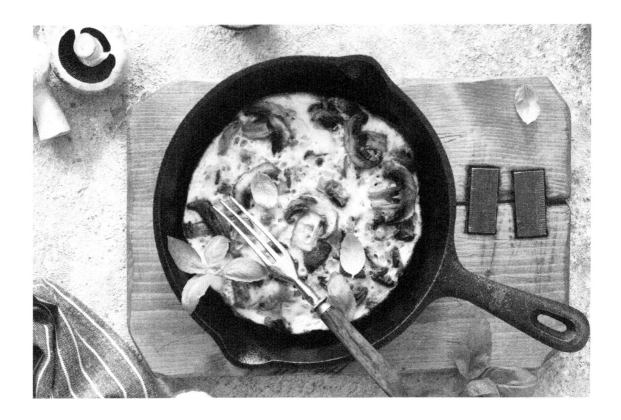

**Makes:** 4 - 5

**Total Prep Time:** 30 Minutes

**Ingredient List:**

- Mushroom (4 cups, shitake, sautéed until softened)
- Eggs (6, large)
- Garlic (1 clove, chopped fine)
- Fontina Cheese (1/4 cup, grated)
- Thyme (1 tablespoon, chopped)
- Skim Milk (1 cup, evaporated)
- Leek (1, finely diced, sautéed until softened)
- Olive oil (1 tsp)
- Salt (1/4 teaspoons)
- Pepper (1/4 teaspoons)
- Cooking spray (enough to coat the pan)

xxxxxxxxxxxxxxxxxxxxxxxxxxxxxxxxxxxxxxxxxxxxxxx

**Procedure:**

A. Preheat the oven to 375°F.
B. In a medium bowl combine your mushrooms and leeks with half of your salt and pepper and olive oil.
C. Spray a pie dish (9 inches) and spoon in your mushroom and leeks spreading to cover the entire bottom of the pie dish.
D. In a bowl mix eggs, garlic, thyme, milk, pepper, and salt then pour the mixture on top of the mushrooms and leeks in your pie dish.
E. Top evenly with fontina cheese. Allow it to bake until puffy and golden in color (about 30 minutes).
F. Allow to cool slightly, serve and enjoy.

# 26. Red Hot Mama Sauce

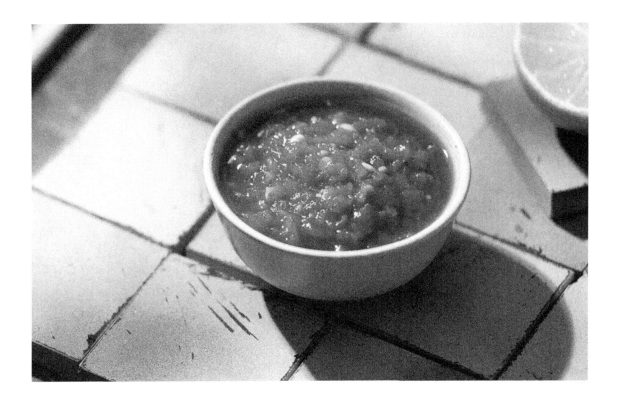

**Makes:** 6

**Total Prep Time:** 7 Minutes

**Ingredient List:**

- Chili paste (1/2 cup)
- Coconut amino (1 tablespoon)
- Mustard (1 teaspoon)
- Stevia (1 teaspoon)

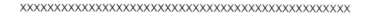

**Procedure:**

A. Add all of your ingredients listedto a large bowl.
B. Stir to combine and enjoy with your selected choice of protein.

# 27. Savory Crepes

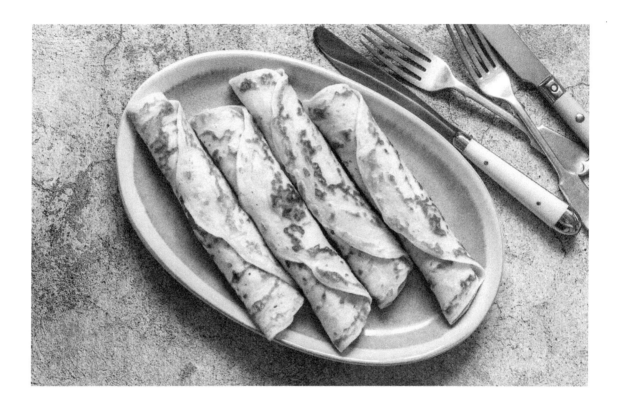

**Makes:** 2

**Total Prep Time:** 15 Minutes

**Ingredient List:**

**Crepes:**

- Eggs (4)
- Almond milk (¼ cup, unsweetened)
- Coconut flour (1 tablespoon)
- Salt (¼ tsp)
- Parsley (¼ cup, finely chopped)
- Coconut oil for frying

**Filling ideas:**

- Avocado (1, peeled, diced)

xxxxxxxxxxxxxxxxxxxxxxxxxxxxxxxxxxxxxxxxxxxxxxx

**Procedure:**

A. Combine all your crepe ingredients listed into a medium bowl, then whisk until a smooth batter is formed.
B. Allow the mixture to stand like this for about 10 minutes to thicken a little.
C. Set a large greased skillet over medium heat to get hot. Stir the batter and add a few tablespoons of the batter to the center of your hot skillet.
D. Swirl the skillet so that the batter spreads and creates a thin layer over the bottom of the skillet. Allow it to cook for about 2 minutes, or until golden brown.
E. Transfer from heat to a serving plate, top with diced avocado, roll, and serve.

# 28. Scrambled Tofu with Smoked Salmon

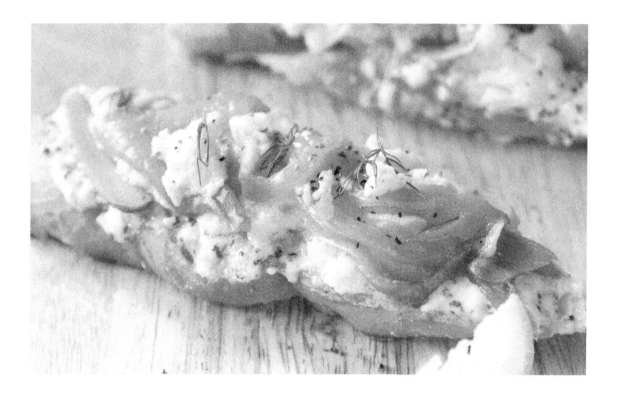

**Makes:** 1

**Total Prep Time:** 15 Minutes

**Ingredient List:**

- Tofu (1/2 lb., firm, crumbled)
- Smoked Salmon (1/8 cup, finely diced)
- Heavy cream (1 tsp)
- Butter (1 tsp)
- Turmeric (1 teaspoon)
- Salt and pepper (2 teaspoons, or to taste)
- Garlic powder (1 tsp)

xxxxxxxxxxxxxxxxxxxxxxxxxxxxxxxxxxxxxxxxxxxxxxxx

**Procedure:**

A. In a small bowl add the tofu, turmeric, garlic powder, and heavy cream then mix around to combine.
B. Over medium heat, melt the butter in a skillet. Pour the tofu mixture into the skillet. Stir constantly.
C. About 5 minutes add in your salmon and continue to stir once the tofu is slightly brown and no longer moist.
D. Add the salt and pepper while it is on the plate.

# 29. Spinach Pesto Egg Muffins

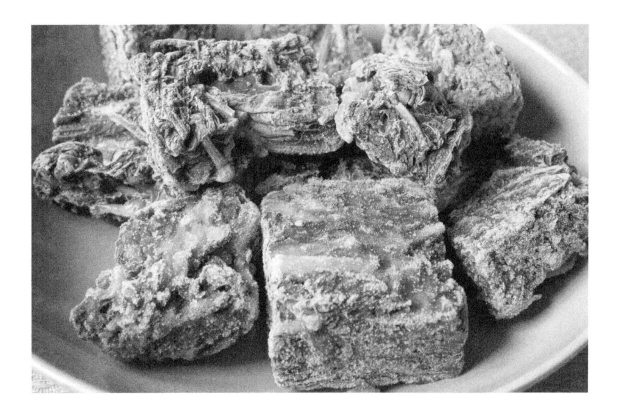

**Makes:** 10

**Total Prep Time:** 30 Minutes

**Ingredient List:**

- Spinach (⅔ cup, frozen, thawed, drained)
- Pesto (3 tablespoons)
- Kalamata olives (½ cup, pitted)
- Sun-dried tomatoes (¼ cup, chopped)
- Goat cheese (125g., soft)
- Eggs (6 large, free-range)
- Salt (to taste)
- Pepper (to taste)

xxxxxxxxxxxxxxxxxxxxxxxxxxxxxxxxxxxxxxxxxxxxxxxxxx

A. **Procedure:**

B. Set your oven to preheat to 350°F and prepare a muffin tin by fitting it with paper muffin cups.

C. Drain as much liquid from your thawed spinach as possible and set aside. Slice olives, and discard seeds then aside. Roughly chop your sun-dried tomatoes.

D. Add your eggs, and pesto into a medium bowl then season to taste with pepper and salt. Whisk until fully combined.

E. Evenly split your olives, chopped tomato, crumbled goat cheese, and spinach between your muffin cups.

F. Top each cup evenly with your pesto egg mixture and set in a preheated oven to bake.

G. Allow to bake until eggs are fully set, and the tops become lightly browned (about 25 minutes).

H. Remove from heat, allow to cool slightly, and serve.

# 30. Grilled Avocado with Melted Cheese Hot Sauce

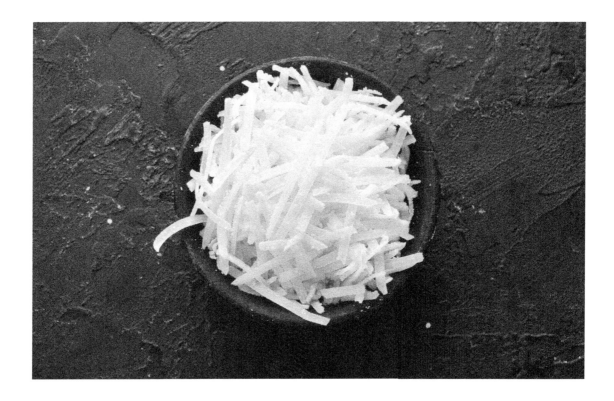

**Makes:** 1

**Total Prep Time:** 9 Minutes

**Ingredient List:**

- Avocado (1)
- Chipotle sauce (1 tablespoon)
- Lime juice (1 tablespoon)
- Parmesan cheese (¼ cup)
- Salt (to taste)
- Pepper (to taste)

xxxxxxxxxxxxxxxxxxxxxxxxxxxxxxxxxxxxxxxxxxxxxxxxx

**Procedure:**

A. Prepare your avocado by slicing it in half lengthwise and discarding the seed.
B. Gently prick the skin of your avocado with a fork randomly and set aside.
C. Set your avocado halves, skin side down, on a small baking sheet, and line them with aluminum foil.
D. Top evenly with your sauce, then drizzle with lime juice. Season to taste with pepper, and salt.
E. Sprinkle half parmesan cheese in each cavity and set your broiler on high for 2 minutes.
F. Add your remaining parmesan cheese, and return to the broiler until the cheese completely melts, and the avocado slightly browns (about another 2 minutes).
G. Serve hot, with a side of extra chipotle sauce.

# Author Biography

Josephine has 4 kids. That means she's a full-time mom who has to cater to difficult flavor requirements and phases sometimes... Her twins don't like mushy foods, her daughter is lactose intolerant, and her son won't eat anything that doesn't have melted nacho cheese on it. In a nutshell, cooking was a nightmare for her. She still did it extremely lovingly, but there's no denying that cooking with so many conditions is difficult. Oh, and let's not forget that cooking for children also requires an art degree because if the food doesn't look fun, inferesting, or yummy there's no way they'll eat it!

At one point, Josephine considered giving in to the frozen food aisle and living off boxed chicken nuggets and frozen lasagna and vegan key-lime pie. However, the thought was quickly chased out of her imagination every time she swiped her card at the supermarket. It was over $350 in groceries every week! She had to do something about it otherwise she'd be broke in a month!

Thus, Josephine started looking into quick and healthy recipes that checked all her children's boxes without breaking the bank either. Within a matter of weeks, her children began to love their mom's home cooking more than ever and even began to open themselves up to new ingredients! After giving it some thought, she decided to start publishing her recipes, hoping to help some moms through picky eating phases and allergies. As long as you don't give in to frozen foods, her recipes will change the way you cook so much you'll actually enjoy it again!

# Author's Afterthoughts

*thank you*

Being a single mother never quite gets "easy", but it's an especially entertaining and complicated feat when they're young. My kiddos are like bouncy balls that have been charged with endless energy. They're here, they're there, they're everywhere! While I have gotten used to all of our adventures, I definitely have to take a moment to thank you for supporting my work.

Not only does it allow me to spend more time with my kids, but it also helps me pay the bills and continue funding new cookbook projects as a single mom. Cooking for my kids during their picky eating phases is always tricky, but thankfully I have you to support me so I can get creative in the kitchen and solve their cravings and your life with all of my recipes.

Just hang in there because it's only a matter of time before my next book comes out, but until then, I'd really like it if you could share your thoughts about my recipes with me. Also, what kind of recipes would you like to see more of? School lunches? Meals for certain allergies? Whatever you come up with will benefit all the moms out there (including myself) who struggle to think of delicious healthy meals our kids will actually eat.

**Keep me posted!**

**Josephine Ellis.**

Printed in Great Britain
by Amazon

21074816R00045